I0476929

Diabetes:

Pain,

Greed and Hope

A personal story!

By

Ray Schenkel

Introduction

This book is for children and young adults to realize how dangerous diabetes is and that it is important to watch your health over and beyond what your doctors tell you. I have been dying from diabetes for nearly 15 years and in telling my story I hope that I may save some lives.

There are nearly 20 million diabetics in the United States today and the number is growing faster and faster every year. There are people and doctors out there who say that diabetes can be prevented. They are flat out lying. You can do things to lesson your chances of getting diabetes such as staying on the thin side and exercising. I can personally say that's bull. I was 5 foot 7 and weighed 160 when I was diagnosed with diabetes. Later in the book we will talk about my friend, Joel Carlson, who was 5 foot 9 and 125 pounds when diagnosed.

Diabetes is hereditary. That means it is passed through family genes or it's a little bug that bites us. Three of my cousins weighed over 400 pounds and guess how many have diabetes: none. The next time you see a doctor on TV saying all the obese Americans are heading for diabetes ignore them. Even if you are thin, you can get diabetes too. My advice to you is if any of your relatives are diabetic you better figure the diabetes will come after you. Many of you may be wondering "what is diabetes?". Diabetes occurs when the sugar levels in your blood become too high and cause problems inside your body. When you eat and drink your body turns the food into glucose which your cells use to make your body work. Your body has an organ called a pancreas that makes insulin so the sugar goes into the cells properly. If your pancreas does not make insulin you have Type 1 Diabetes. If your pancreas doesn't make enough insulin or it's not working properly with your cells, you have Type 2 diabetes. Type 2 is the kind of diabetes that 90% of the people have and the type this book is about.

My Story

I was around 41 when I went to the doctor to get a blood test so I could go to North Carolina to teach. While I'm there, the doctor said, "We should measure your cholesterol". I said, "Why not?"

I went back to work at an office supply store I owned in Ada, Minnesota. That night I went to visit my Mom and help her to bed since she had a lung infection and was very ill. I had been taking care of her since she had heart attack the year before.

The next morning I get a call from the clinic to come over and get a blood test. The doctor came in and said, "Your blood test indicates that you have diabetes. On an A1C chart you tested at a 9.9." He continued to say that I should be put on insulin that I can inject daily. The doctor thought for a moment and then said, "We can start you out on this pill called Metformin." I took it for a week and all it did was cause me to have diarrhea all the time. This prompted me to do research and I discovered the Atkins diet for diabetes. Within a week, my sugar numbers were going down like a rocket. It was a hard diet to follow but I did it for two weeks. After the two weeks, I went back to the doctor and said, "Test my blood again". The doctor said it would be a waste of time. We just tested you a short while ago. I insisted that we test it that day. We did. It came back at 6.9 on the A1C chart. The doctor said that I starved myself. I told him no, I just eliminated my carbohydrates. He then said that whatever I do I need to make sure that my A1C stays under 7.0.

After that, I came back every year and had my A1C checked to see if it was staying in line. I also had an eye exam every year because the diabetic bug loves your eyes. Eyes have small arteries and veins that diabetes can ruin. It is very important to get everything checked once a year.

Doctors will tell you over and over nothing on Earth can stop diabetes. For the next several years my diabetes was napping or planning. During the year of 2014, my blood pressure started to climb above normal to 150/80.   My A1C was 7.3 which is a fair number. My eye doctor was continuously telling me that my blood pressure had to be lowered. My regular doctor prescribed Lisinopril. Come to find out, that drug might have been the first prescribed drug to damage my kidneys. In the summer, I went to my eye doctor in Minnesota. He then called my regular doctor in North Carolina and informed him that they need to do some emergency work on my blood pressure to save my eyes.

The minute I get back to North Carolina I saw my doctor. He changed my blood pressure medications. At that time he also got me on a referral list to see a kidney specialist in Greensboro. Three months later I see Dr. C, the kidney specialist. That first day he told me my kidneys were in real trouble and prescribed some pills. What a disaster! Two days later my whole body was covered in blisters. I discovered that I am allergic to the medicine. Two more days later I am sent to a skin doctor where they cut off the blisters. In July, I had a kidney biopsy done and found out that my kidneys were not functioning well enough due to high blood pressure and diabetes.

I started the school year, but in October I had to go on a leave of absence. I stopped teaching and went on dialysis. Ironically, in the seven months that I was with my kidney doctor not once did he try anything to slow the progress of my kidney failure.   All he did was prescribe some other high blood pressure medications and one specifically, Benicar, made my kidneys fail faster.

People say that dialysis is like death or worse. I can't say that but it is a very unpleasant experience. There are two types of dialysis. You can go to a center where blood is taken out of your body for four hours, filtered for toxins, and then pumped back into your body.   A dialysis center is like a waiting room for the funeral home. The people are without hope and look worse due to diabetes, i.e., no feet, blind, can't stand or walk. The other type of dialysis is peritoneal dialysis (PD) which you do at home. In this endeavor, a machine called the cycler pumps fluid in and out of your abdomen for 10 hours using the fill, dwell and drain routine.

First, I was on Hemo dialysis at a center so I had a catheter put through in the veins in my chest to my heart. It does not hurt but it is strange to have two tubes sticking out of your chest. The worst thing about Hemo dialysis is that you feel so tired all the time. I also got extreme headaches that would not go away even with medications. You can hardly live your life.

Next, I got a catheter placed in my stomach so I could do PD dialysis at home. They forgot to put a cap on tightly and it fell off and exposed my insides to bacteria. As a result, I developed a massive infection called peritonitis. I went on an antibiotic regime to get rid of this infection which is very difficult to get rid of. During this time, the catheter got stuck in my lower abdomen.   Two days later I am in a Raleigh hospital to have surgery to move, and then tack the catheter in place so it won't get stuck again. For a month, I was on intervenious antibiotics to save me and with God's help, I made it.

At the same time the diabetes attacked my kidneys, it went after my eyes. The blood vessels in my retinas began to break open and my vision went blurry and dysfunctional. My vision now is a lot better. Over the last several months, I had two laser eye surgeries. Seven times they had to use a needle to put medicine in the back of my eyes. The laser and the needles are not as painful as you would think but they are scary to go through. In the future I will have to get these procedures repeated several times. When you have diabetes, your health can turn bad and it seems like every day another part of your body goes bad. I have not mentioned all things that have happened to me such as unexplained pains, body temperature, and rashes.

In case you ever get this terrible disease, please watch your own numbers, get tested for everything every six months to make sure nothing major is going wrong, especially your kidney function and your eyes.

Doctor, Doctor

In this world there are some great doctors and some crappy ones, but most fall somewhere in between. I think most people place too much faith in their doctors; probably because this is the traditional society norm. Many of our medical doctors are too complacent and write too many prescriptions. They fail to ask the "why" question. They are so quick to prescribe medicine for symptoms rather then ask why the patient has the problem.

This is most evident with diabetes. In the fifteen years that I have had diabetes not one doctor will see what is causing my diabetes.   Is it the pancreas... it doesn't make insulin or my cells don't process sugar properly? Anyone who has diabetes call tell you about a typical doctor's visit where everything that is wrong with you is diabetes. I swear if they know you have diabetes all rational thinking goes out the window. If I went to my regular doctor with an arrow in my chest and I asked what he thought what was wrong he would say if you didn't have diabetes you would have been able to duck quicker. This is an exaggeration but those of you that have diabetes know this is not that far from the truth. When you have diabetes, it becomes the cause of all your health problems.

Most doctors don't do a good job of putting themselves in a patient's shoes with diabetes. The patient is usually surprised, scared and confused. They don't feel bad and yet they face a lifetime of problems. Diabetes is like a lifetime prison sentence with no chance for parole. You can try to control it but you are never really in charge as diabetes can rear its head in many ways. The only sure end is death.

Doctors like to say you can control it and live a long life. This is true for some, but not for all. Because of their authoritative role, many doctors speak before they think and misconceptions occur. Here are some examples of things that doctors have said to me in the past year. A physician's assistant at my regular doctor's office had not seen me in a few months. When I came in for a visit she said, "I thought you would be dead by now." That was a lot better than good morning.

Another physician's assistant that I was seeing at another clinic said the following when I was asking him about the medications that I was taking for my high blood pressure and I was wondering if he had any ideas to help. He said, "Take more "sleeping pills" it will lower your blood pressure."

The best was a doctor at a kidney transplant center who said, "You should hope to get liver cancer and then you will put on the top of the list for both a kidney and liver transplant." I have never heard of anybody being told to wish for a terminal condition. Why did they say these things? I think they feel obligated to have an answer. Like everyone else, doctors are pressured by time and money.

Money kills Cure

There is no disease that won't be cured for the same reason as diabetes. The drug companies won't allow it. They would kill anybody who got close to a cure. Drug companies make more money off of diabetes than any other illness in the world. In fact, their greed even stops some of the innovation. There are hundreds of companies making a fortune off diabetics from alcohol pads, lancets to medications and dialysis machines. They love that diabetics live for years and keep coming back for more supplies and drugs. This concept is a money windfall.

Let's start with the small and build our way up. The most basic thing a diabetic does is check their blood sugar.   They use a lancet or needle to poke their finger to draw blood which they put on a test strip then place that strip into a glucose meter. The manufacturers of these items make a fortune using the following method. Only their lancets work in their holders. Their test strips only work in their meters eliminating any competition. They also lure people in by pricing the meters cheap and then the test strips are outrageously high priced. A pack of a hundred test strips can be well over a hundred dollars. It is ridiculous when you realize these pieces of thick paper are made by the millions for less than a cent a piece. It is not like this is new technology. Meters and strips have remained the same for over twenty years. The most ironic thing is why blood sugar levels are taken this way. When you go to the hospital the first thing they do is put a clip on your finger that measures your pulse and the oxygen content in your blood. If you can read oxygen content through the skin, why not sugar? The reason is it would put the strip and meter business into the dust bin of history and we are talking about a lot of money. There is no way this technology is beyond our grasps today. We can scan blood flow inside the heart yet we can't scan blood for sugar.

Next is insulin, the drug many diabetics are treated with on a daily basis. We have been manufacturing insulin for over fifty years and unlike any other commodity the price hasn't come down. For some bottles of insulin the price is well over two hundred dollars and in most cases the company spends more on the packaging than the product. It doesn't take any new research to make insulin. This has been known for decades thus these companies are plain greedy and love to price gouge.

Worst of all, the drugs for diabetes are often very similar. About every week a new one comes out and it is nearly exactly like the one that was made ten years earlier. They change one little part then patent them as new and price to the max. In fact the only drug that does work is metformin and it was invented eighty years ago. All diabetic drugs have side effects that are nearly worse than the diabetes.

With severe diet changes most people could realize benefits as good as these drugs without the risks. Dr. Atkins proved that twenty years ago with no carbs, no sugar. It is just too hard to stay on a super low carb diet. Lastly, is the dialysis you have to have when your kidneys fail. Dialysis or death are your options. After seven months on dialysis I am not sure I picked the right option. Many years ago the US Congress made it that any person on dialysis was put on Medicare. That is why we have dialysis centers today because no person could afford it. When the government did this they created an industry that most people in the country know nothing about. There are several of these billion dollar companies around the country. They own the dialysis machines, the kidney doctors and nurses, plus other side groups such as drug makers, food vendors, and other types of special doctors. It all begins when a diabetic's kidneys start to fail. They get sent to a kidney specialist who gets them into their dialysis center and on the companies' supplies. In my opinion, from the first day forward the kidney doctor and the dialysis company have two things in common. They have the need to make millions of dollars and keep that dialysis patient alive and on dialysis. The patient is now a cash cow. The patient's health or chance of getting better is totally irrelevant. The only concern is that he/she survives for as long as possible. This is why most dialysis patients have so little hope. The only thing they look forward to is a visit by the grim reaper. While on dialysis, many patients will lose limbs and their eye sight yet their kidney doctor or the company will have little concern. Their goal is to keep the patient alive and attached to the machine so the money flows in. That's their passion.

Make it Better

What can we do to make this better? I am going to start an organization called the Diabetic Hope Group. Its goal will be to shine some light on the practices mentioned in this book. If the government and general public knew of some these things, they might change their policies. There are twenty million diabetics in this country and if we spoke as one, things would change. We want a cure, not another set of copycat drugs. Twenty years ago, the British cloned a whole sheep and I am sure the copy had working organs inside it. Why can't we take a sample of a person's pancreas and use the working parts to clone a new one. There would be no question of matching. This sounds like a complex concept but think what Sauk and Pasteur did with little to no equipment or money. We have all this technology today, spend billions and nothing gets solved. This may be the time to use a conservative method with all the researchers every year. Show us what you've got or your funds get cut to zero. You will see some action then; I guarantee it!

Charts on Diabetes and Dialysis

Affected, where they live, drug companies, race and gender.

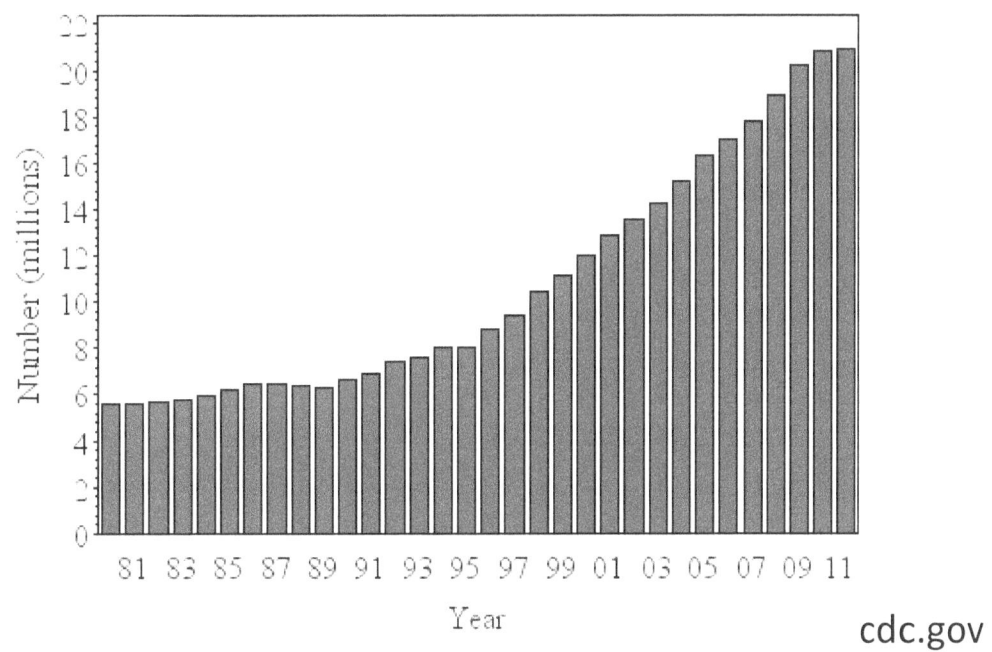

cdc.gov

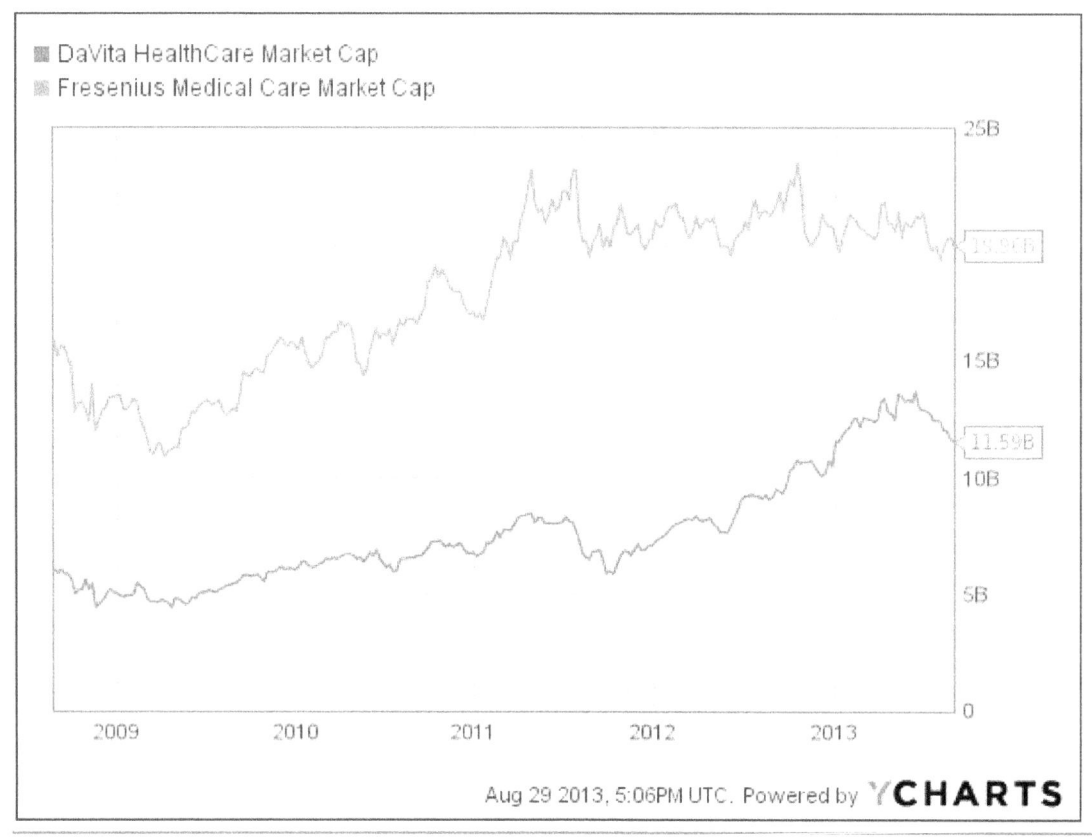

- DaVita HealthCare Market Cap
- Fresenius Medical Care Market Cap

25B

15B

11.59B

10B

5B

0

2009   2010   2011   2012   2013

Aug 29 2013, 5:06PM UTC. Powered by YCHARTS

Waiting for a kidney

Although 6 percent of Wisconsin's population is black, African Americans make up 26.1 percent of the waiting list.

White
Population 85%
Waiting 58.6%

Black
Population 6%
Waiting 26.1%

Hispanic
Population 5%
Waiting 6.9%

Asian
Population 2%
Waiting 6.6%

Other
Population 2%
Waiting 2.1%*

NOTE: Population is based on 2008 figures.

* Includes multi-racial

SOURCE: United Network for Organ Sharing; U.S. Census Bureau

The Capital Times

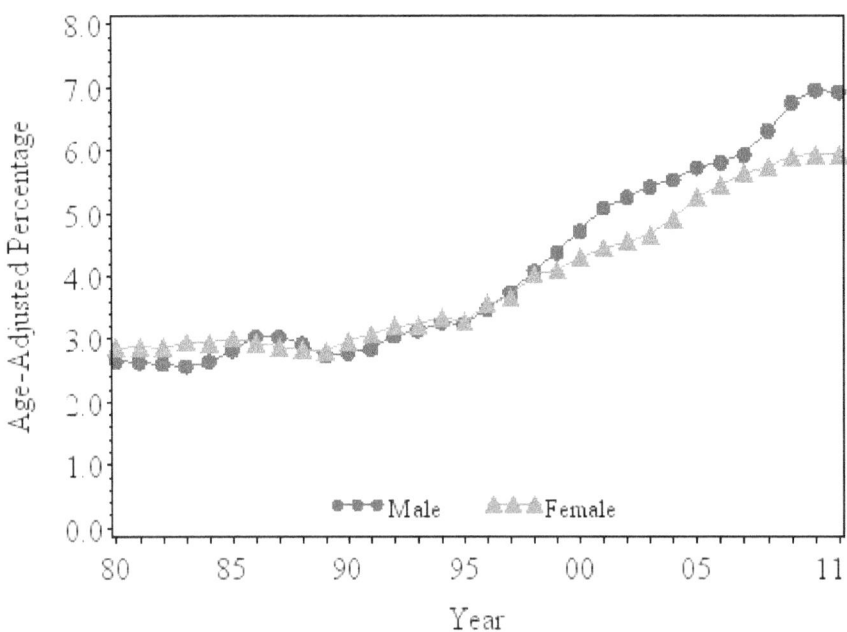

What American Diabetes Association gets paid by Drug Companies

It equals 19 million year.

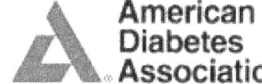

2008 Revenues Received By the American Diabetes Association

Company	Donations (Includes Contributions, Sponsorships and (Grants)	Fees From Transactions (Includes Advertising, Exhibiting and Book Sales)	Total Revenue
Abbott/Abbott Diabetes Care	$597,964	$515,075	$1,113,039
Amylin Pharmaceuticals	$704,500	$140,910	$1,114,860
AstraZeneca	$73,437	$0	$73,437
AstraZeneca/Bristol Myers Squibb	$203,635	$114,450	$318,085
Bayer HealthCare	$95,949	$408,613	$504,562
BD Diabetes	$315,391	$398,895	$714,286
Boehringer-Ingelheim Pharmaceuticals	$150,000	$116,000	$266,000
Bristol Myers-Squibb Company	$140,198	$114,450	$254,648
Eli Lilly and Company	$778,300	$665,288	$1,443,588
GlaxoSmithKline	$432,400	$92,120	$524,520
LifeScan Inc.	$144,704	$175,047	$319,751

Here is why there will never be cure

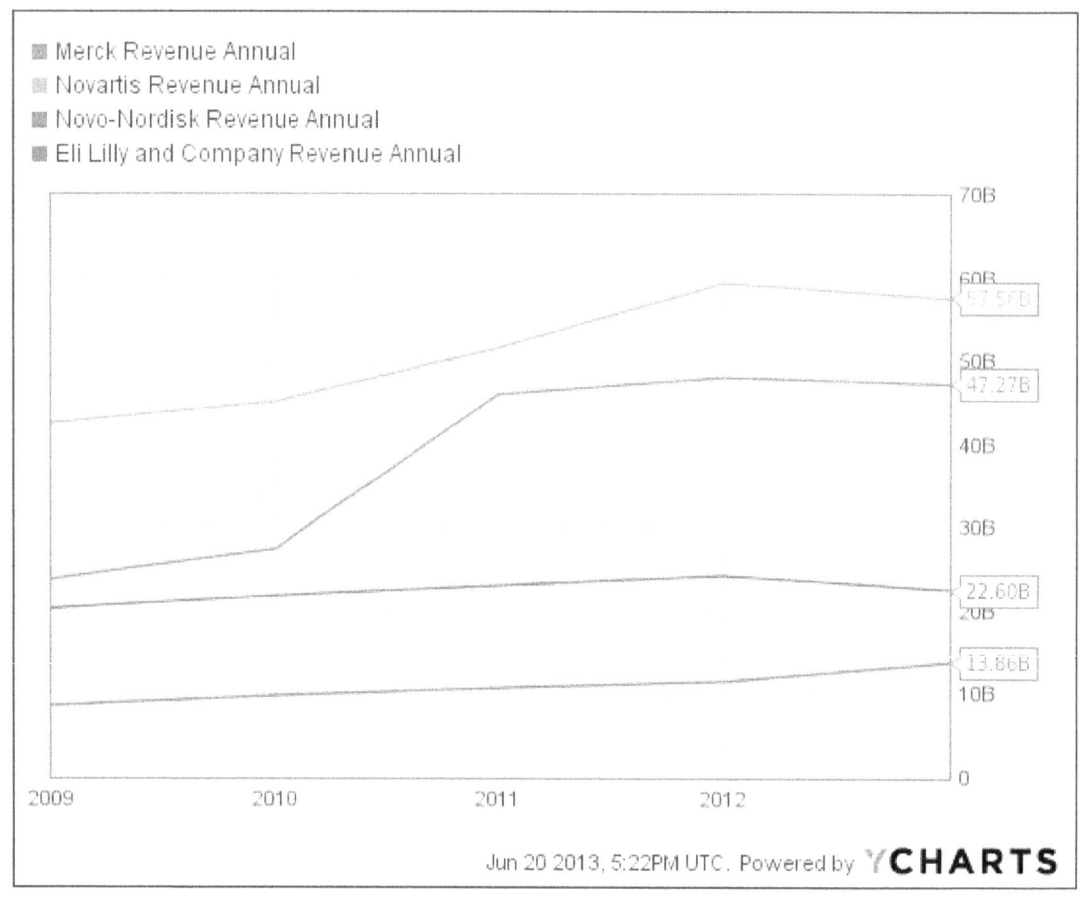

.

Diabetes Glossary

Diabetes A to Z

A1C - A blood test that measures average blood glucose over the past 2 to 3 months and is the best way to measure overall glucose control. It should be measured 2 to 4 times a year and the goal is less than 7%.

Acanthosis nigricans - a thickening and darkening of the skin in patchy areas in the skin folds of the armpits, neck, or groin, ranging from tan to dark brown. This is usually a sign of insulin resistance.

ACE inhibitor (angiotensin-converting enzyme) - a type of medication used to lower blood pressure and help treat kidney problems related to diabetes.

Adult stem cell - a cell found in the different tissues of the body – such as blood, skin or muscle – that can renew itself and produce the specialized cells needed by that tissue (known as multipotency).

Antibodies - proteins that the body makes to protect itself from foreign substances such as bacteria and viruses.

ARBs (angiotensin receptor blocker) - a type of oral medication used to lower blood pressure.

Atherosclerosis - a process that involves thickening of the blood vessel walls thought to be related to inflammation of the vessel wall, which then leads to formation of plaques, causing partial blockages. If these plaques rupture, clots form on that rupture site, causing a more acute, total blockage. If the blood vessel is providing blood to the heart, the result would be a heart attack.

Autoimmune disease - disorder of the body's immune system in which the immune system mistakenly attacks and destroys body tissue considered foreign.

Basal insulin - the insulin that controls blood glucose levels between meals and overnight. It controls glucose in the fasting state.

Beta cells - cells that produce insulin. They are located within the islets of Langerhans in the pancreas.

Blood glucose (or glucose) - a type of sugar that is created when the carbohydrate that one eats is broken down in the body. During digestion, glucose passes through the wall of the intestine into the bloodstream to the liver and eventually into the general circulation. From there glucose can then enter individual cells or tissues throughout the body to be used for fuel and provide energy.

Blood pressure - the pressure against the walls of your blood vessels. High blood pressure is more common in persons with diabetes and increases the risk of stroke, heart attack, kidney and eye diseases. It should be measured at every doctor visit, or at least once a year, with a goal of 130/80 mm Hg or lower.

Body mass index (BMI)- a method of determining by the relationship between height and weight whether or not a person is obese, overweight, underweight or of normal weight.

Bolus insulin - the insulin that is released when food is eaten. A *bolus* is a burst of insulin that is delivered by injection or by the insulin pump to "cover" a meal or snack or to correct for a high blood glucose level.

Carbohydrate counting - a meal planning method commonly used by people with diabetes to plan their food and meal choices. Carbohydrate counting helps one achieve a balance between the amount of carbohydrate foods eaten and the available insulin.

Carbohydrate - the main source of fuel for the body. Carbohydrate includes starches and sugars and are found in bread, pasta, fruits, vegetables, milk, and sweets. Carbs are broken down into a sugar called *glucose.*

Cardiologist - a doctor who specializes in the heart and vascular system.

Cardiovascular system - the heart and blood vessels. It is the means by which blood is pumped from the heart and circulated throughout the body. As it circulates, the blood carries nourishment and oxygen to all of the body's tissues. It also removes waste products.

Charcot foot - a condition in which the small bones of the foot become misaligned, leading to foot deformity. It is a problem that can evolve as a result of nerve damage.

Cholesterol - a type of fat that is manufactured in the liver or intestines, but is also found in some of the foods we eat. (Only animal foods, such as eggs, milk, cheese, liver, meat and poultry contain cholesterol).

Clinical trials - carefully controlled studies that are conducted to test the effectiveness and safety of new drugs, medical products or techniques. All drugs in the U.S. undergo three phases of clinical trials before being approved for general use.

Cloning - a process for creating a genetically identical copy of a cell or an organism.

Conventional insulin therapy - an insulin therapy in which the insulin regimen is decided first and the person with diabetes has to eat and engage in physical activity according to the time actions of the injected insulins.

Creatinine - a waste product derived from the activity of the muscles. Normally, kidneys can remove this substance from the blood. A buildup of creatinine in the blood signals that the kidneys are losing their ability to function normally.

Dawn phenomenon - a rise in blood glucose levels that occurs in the early morning hours.

Diabetes educator - a healthcare person who has the skill and knowledge to teach a person with diabetes how to manage the condition. Diabetes educators may be doctors, nurses, dietitians, mental health or fitness clinicians.   Some also have the credential CDE (Certified Diabetes Educator).

Diabetic ketoacidosis (also called **ketoacidosis or DKA**) - a condition that results from a lack of sufficient insulin in the body, leading to high blood glucose levels and ketone formation. It is an extremely serious and life-threatening condition that may lead to coma and death. The symptoms of ketoacidosis are nausea, stomach pain, vomiting, chest pain, rapid shallow breathing, and difficulty staying awake.

Diabetic macular edema - a condition that can occur in either stage of diabetic retinopathy (nonproliferative retinopathy, and a more serious stage called proliferative retinopathy) in which fluid collects in the central part of the retina resulting in blurred vision. Macular edema can be treated with laser surgery when central vision is threatened.

Differentiation - the process by which an unspecialized cell changes into a more organized or complex cell that performs a certain function, such as an insulin-producing beta cell.

Embryonic stem cell - an unspecialized cell in an embryo that can divide indefinitely (self renew) and produce any cell in the body needed after birth (known as pluripotency).

Endocrinologist - a doctor who specializes in diseases of the endocrine system such as diabetes.

Epidemiology - the study of disease patterns in human populations.

Fasting blood glucose test - a blood test in which a sample of your blood is drawn after an overnight fast to measure the amount of glucose in your blood.

Fructosamine test-a blood test that can detect overall changes in blood glucose control over a shorter time-span than the A1C test. Fructosamine levels indicate the level of blood glucose control over the past two or three weeks. Thus, when rapid changes are being made in your diabetes treatment plan, this test quickly tells you how the changes are working and whether other changes should be considered.

Gastroparesis - a condition in which neuropathy affects the nerves controlling the digestive tract and causes difficulty processing or disposing of food. It can cause nausea, vomiting, bloating or diarrhea.

Gestational diabetes - diabetes that develops during pregnancy. During this time, some women will have only a minimal insulin deficiency and will be able to adequately control their blood glucose with a meal plan. Other women may have a more severe insulin deficiency and require insulin along with nutrition therapy to control their blood glucose. This type of diabetes usually lasts only through the pregnancy, but women who have it may be at greater risk of developing type 2 diabetes later on.

Ghrelin - a hormone that relays messages between the digestive system and the brain. It works to stimulate appetite, slow metabolism, and decrease your body's ability to burn fat.

Glucose - a simple form of sugar that is created when the body's digestive processes break down the food we eat. Glucose is the body's main source of energy.

Glucose meter - a device that measures one's blood glucose levels.

Glucose tolerance test - blood test done every hour or at the 2-hour point after drinking a sugar-filled liquid. This is one test used to diagnose diabetes. If at 2 hours, your blood glucose rises to over 200 mg/dl you have diabetes. This test is not as common as a fasting glucose test.

Glycemic index **(GI)** - a system of ranking foods containing equal amounts of carbohydrate according to how much they raise blood glucose levels. For instance, the carbohydrate in a slice of 100% stone-ground whole wheat bread (a low glycemic index food) may have less impact on blood glucose than a slice of processed white bread (a high glycemic index food). The GI is an additional meal-planning tool to help one understand how carbohydrate foods can differ in their effects on blood glucose.

Glycemic load (GL) - a system of ranking carbohydrate foods based on how much they raise blood glucose levels that combines the GI value and the carbohydrate content of an average serving of a food, of a meal, or of a day's worth of food.

Glycogen - glucose that is stored in muscles and liver.

HDL (high-density lipoprotein—also called "**good" cholesterol**) - a type of blood cholesterol that sweeps excess cholesterol from the blood back to the liver where it is reprocessed or eliminated.

Health services - services performed by health care professionals or by others under their direction for the purpose of promoting, maintaining, or restoring health.

Hormones - chemical messengers made in one part of the body to transfer "information" through the bloodstream to cells in another part of the body. Insulin is a hormone.

Hyperglycemia - high blood glucose levels. Blood glucose is generally considered "high" when it is 160 mg/dl or above your individual blood glucose target.

Hyperosmolar hyperglycemic state (HHS) - a serious condition resulting from extremely high levels of blood glucose, causing excessive urination and severe dehydration, but without ketones. It is not very common.

Hypertension - high blood pressure (blood flows through the blood vessels with a greater than normal force) which is defined as blood pressure equal to or greater than 140/90 mm Hg and affects the majority of adults with diabetes. It increases one's risk of heart attack, stroke and kidney problems.

Hypoglycemia - a blood glucose below 80 mg/dl with or without symptoms or below 90 mg/dl with symptoms.

Hypoglycemia unawareness - a condition in which one no longer recognizes the symptoms of low blood glucose.

Impaired fasting glucose (IFG) - a fasting glucose level between 100 mg/dl and 125 mg/dl. Fasting blood test results between these levels mean that you have pre-diabetes.

Impaired glucose tolerance (IGT) - a blood glucose level after a 2-hour glucose tolerance test between 140 and 199 mg/dl. This means you have pre-diabetes.

Infusion set - plastic tubing used with an insulin pump.

Insulin - a hormone made in the pancreas that helps glucose pass into the cells where it is used to create energy for the body.

Insulin pen - an insulin delivery method that looks like a writing pen.

Insulin reaction (hypoglycemia) - low blood glucose resulting from either too much insulin, too much activity or too little food.

Insulin resistance - a condition that makes it harder for the cells to properly use insulin.

Insulin pump - an insulin delivery system; a small mechanical device, typically the size of a beeper or small cell phone, that releases insulin into the tissues of the body by way of tubing and a needle.

Insulin sensitivity factor (also called the **correction factor** or **supplemental factor**) - the amount of blood glucose measured in mg/dl that is lowered by 1 unit of rapid-acting or regular insulin. The insulin sensitivity factor is used to calculate the amount of insulin you need to return blood glucose to within your target blood glucose range.

Insulin-to-carbohydrate ratio - a method of determining how much rapid-acting insulin is needed to cover the carbohydrate eaten at a meal or snack. This is used as part of a more advanced level of carbohydrate counting.

Islet cells - cells that make insulin and are found within the pancreas; also called pancreatic beta cells.

Islet cell transplantation - transplanting islet beta cells that produce insulin from a donor pancreas into a person whose pancreas no longer produces insulin.

Islets of Langerhans - cells found in the pancreas, the most important of which are *beta cells*– the tiny factories that make insulin.

Intermediate-acting insulin- a type of insulin that begins to work to lower blood glucose within 1 to 4 hours and works hardest 4 to 15 hours after injection. The intermediate-acting insulins are NPH and lente.

Ketones - acids produced due to lack of enough insulin to use the glucose in your bloodstream. Your body turns to its fat stores for energy. When this occurs, ketones are produced, which accumulate in the blood and spill into the urine. These ketones are made when fat is metabolized as a source of energy. The excessive formation of ketones in the blood is called *ketosis,* and the presence of ketones in the urine is called *ketonuria.*Allowed to go untreated, the combination of high blood glucose and ketones can lead to *ketoacidosis (also called DKA).*

Ketonuria - the presence of ketones in the urine.

Ketosis - the excessive formation of ketones in the blood.

Lancet - a small needle used to get a drop of blood from your finger, arm, or other site. The blood is placed on a special strip, which is put into the meter. The meter "reads" the strip and gives a blood glucose reading.

Lifestyle changes - changes made to one's eating habits and physical activity in order to control blood glucose.

Long-acting peaking- a type of insulin that doesn't begin to work to lower blood glucose until 4 to 6 hours after injection It works hardest from 8 to 30 hours after injection and continues to work for up to 24 to 36 hours. The long-acting peaking insulin is ultralente.

Long-acting peakless- a type of basal insulin that begins to work to lower blood glucose within one to two hours after injection and works for 24 hours. The long-acting peakless insulin is glargine.

Lymphocytes - immune system cells that identify and destroy foreign agents such as viruses, bacteria and parasites.

LDL (low-density lipoprotein) - a type of blood cholesterol that is considered "bad" because it can be deposited in the arteries, increasing the risk of heart attack or stroke.

.

Medical nutrition therapy - a method of controlling blood glucose by working with a dietitian to assess one's food and nutrition needs and then developing and following an individualized meal plan.

Mediterranean-type diet - a type of eating plan that is low in saturated fat and cholesterol, high in fruits, vegetables, nuts and grains and that also emphasizes controlling portion sizes to help in reducing overall calories.

Metabolic syndrome -a cluster of conditions that increase the risk of developing vascular disease (heart disease, strokes, and peripheral vascular disease). The most recognizable components of this syndrome are abdominal obesity, high blood pressure (hypertension), high triglycerides (part of the lipid profile), low HDL (the "good" cholesterol) and glucose intolerance.

Metabolism - the process by which the cells of the body change food so that it can be used for energy or so that it can be used to build or maintain cells and tissues.

Microalbumin test - a urine test that measures the presence of small amounts of a protein called albumin.

Microalbuminuria - the presence of small amounts of albumin, a protein, in the urine. Microalbuminuria is an early sign of kidney damage.

Mixed dose - an injection that contains two or more types of insulin given in the same syringe at the same time.

Necrobiosis lipoidica diabeticorum (NLD) - a skin condition believed to result from inflammation of the skin in which the skin thins out, becoming discolored and dimpled. This is the most specific skin problem among people with diabetes. It can be quite disfiguring.

Nephrologist - a doctor who specializes in conditions of the kidney.

Nephropathy - serious kidney disease that can occur in people who have had diabetes for a long time, particularly if their diabetes has been poorly controlled.

Neurologist - a doctor who specializes in conditions of the nervous system.

Neuropathy - damage to the nerves. It is a condition that can be very debilitating and painful. There are two main types of neuropathy, depending on which nerve cells are damaged. One type is called *sensory neuropathy,* which affects feelings in the legs or hands and is referred to as peripheral neuropathy. The other type is*autonomic neuropathy,* which affects nerves that control various organs, such as the stomach or urinary tract.

Nocturnal hypoglycemia - low blood glucose that occurs in the middle of the night.

Noncaloric or nonnutritive sweeteners - sweeteners that contribute few, if any calories and have no effect on blood glucose levels.

Nonproliferative retinopathy - the initial stage in diabetic retinopathy. High levels of blood glucose cause damage to the blood vessels in the retina. The blood vessels leak fluid, which can collect and cause the retina to swell.

Nutritive or caloric sweeteners - sweeteners that contribute calories and can affect blood glucose levels.

Ophthalmologist - a doctor specializing in conditions of the eyes.

Oral glucose-lowering medications (also referred to as **oral antidiabetes medications**) - "diabetes pills," which are used in combination with a meal plan and physical activity as well as in combination with each other and sometimes with insulin to control blood glucose levels.

Outcomes - results, impacts or consequences.

Pancreas - a small gland located below and just behind the stomachthat makes a specific kind of hormone called insulin.

Pathophysiology - changes that occur within an organ or tissue due to disease.

Physiologic insulin therapy (also called **intensive insulin therapy**) - an insulin program that attempts to provide insulin in the way that your body would if you didn't have diabetes. Insulin is adjusted to accommodate your food intake and your activity level, and as a result insulin doses change from one day to the next.

Physiology - the study of the physical and chemical processes involved in the functioning of the human body.

Pre-diabetes - a condition in which either your fasting or two-hour post-meal blood glucose levels are higher than normal, but not high enough for a diagnosis of type 2 diabetes. Studies show that most people with pre-diabetes will develop type 2 diabetes within 10 years if they don't change their lifestyle. They also have a higher risk of developing cardiovascular disease.

Proliferative retinopathy - a more serious stage of diabetic retinopathy in which there is a greater loss of vision or even total blindness. During this stage, abnormal blood vessels grow over the surface of the retina.

Protein - one of the main nutrients from food along with carbohydrate and fat. The body uses protein to build and repair body tissue. Muscles, organs, bones, skin, and many of the hormones in the body are made from protein. As a secondary role, protein can also provide energy for the body if carbohydrate is not available. Food sources of protein include meat, poultry, fish, eggs, dairy products and beans.

Rapid-acting insulin - a type of insulin that begins to work to lower blood glucose within 10 to 30 minutes and works hardest 30 minutes to 3 hours after injection. There are three approved rapid-acting insulins: lispro, aspart and glulisine.

Rebound hyperglycemia (high blood glucose or the Somogyi phenomenon)- a condition in which, as a result of too low a level of glucose, the counterregulatory or stress hormones cause the liver to release too much glucose.

Regenerative medicine - therapies using stem cells to replace or repair damaged or defective tissue.

Regular - the common form of short-acting insulin.

Relative insulin deficiency - a decline in insulin production, which is usually a problem with or without insulin resistanceearly on in the course of diabetes.

Retina - the thin, light-sensitive inner lining in the back of your eye.

Retinopathy - damage to the *retina,* the thin, light-sensitive inner lining in the back of the eye. This damage occurs to small blood vessels in the retina which are easily harmed by high levels of glucose in the blood.

Saturated fat - a type of food fat that is solid at room temperature. Saturated fats raise blood cholesterol levels by interfering with the entry of cholesterol into cells causing cholesterol to remain in the bloodstream longer and to become a part of the plaque that builds up in the blood vessels.

Self-monitoring - managing one's diabetes by checking blood glucose, and being aware of food intake, physical activity and medication and how each of these elements work together in order to keep blood glucose in good control.

SMBG (self-monitoring of blood glucose) - checking your blood glucose with a blood glucose meter.

Short-acting insulin- a type of insulin that begins to work to lower blood glucose within 30 to 60 minutes and works hardest 1 to 5 hours after injection. The common form of short-acting insulin is called *regular*.

Single dose - an injection that contains one type of insulin.

Sugar alcohols or polyols - sweeteners that replace other sugars in foods causing slightly lower rises in blood glucose.

Trans fats - a type of fat formed from *hydrogenation,* a chemical process that changes a liquid oil into a solid fat. Trans fats are found in processed foods, such as snack foods, cookies, fast foods, and some stick or solid margarines. They can raise cholesterol levels and should be eaten in as small amounts as possible.

Triglycerides - a type of fat stored in fat cells as body fat and burned for energy. High levels of triglycerides are linked with an increased risk of heart and blood vessel disease.

Unsaturated fat (both *polyunsaturated* and *monounsaturated*) - fats that comes primarily from vegetables and are liquid at room temperature. Polyunsaturated fats can help lower cholesterol levels. Monounsaturated fats also help lower blood cholesterol levels and may help to raise HDL cholesterol levels.

Vitrectomy surgery - a process to remove the blood and scar tissue from within the eye that can frequently successfully restore vision.

If a Doctor uses a word about your diabetic condition you should find it here. This glossary is from Joslin Diabetes web site.